Comfor

GASTRITIS
MANAGEMENT

Nutrition-Packed Recipes
for Gut Wellness

BY

KENNETH J. MCNAMEE

COMFORT AND HEALING FOR GASTRITIS MANAGEMENT

Nutrition-Packed Recipes for Gut Wellness

First Edition, 2024

Printed In the United States of America

DISCLAIMER

This book is intended for informational purposes only and is not a substitute for professional medical advice, diagnosis, or treatment. The author is not a licensed medical professional. Always seek the advice of your physician or other qualified health provider with any questions you may have regarding a medical condition.

magine a cookbook that serves as a comforting embrace on a plate—nutritious and delectable. That's the vision driving this cookbook. With compassion and understanding, I extend a supportive hand to those navigating the challenges of gastritis, offering nourishment through simple yet satisfying meals. Having personally experienced the pain and discomfort of stomach issues, I empathize with the frustration of being sidelined by intense pain, immobilized, and waiting for relief. It underscores the profound impact of food choices on our well-being. By embracing wholesome, disciplined eating habits, regardless of age, you're not just indulging in good taste but also nurturing your body toward healing. This cookbook aims to illuminate a path toward improved health and vitality, one delicious recipe at a time.

This book is dedicated to Mike - JS.
A great friend, a lifelong mentor
and the best roommate ever!

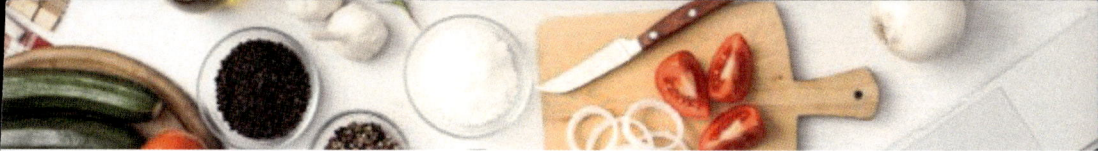

CONTENTS

INTRODUCTION

Embracing Wholesome Gastritis Management

Welcome to a culinary journey crafted with care for those seeking comfort and balance while managing gastritis. In these pages, you'll discover a collection of nurturing recipes designed to support digestive health without compromising flavor or satisfaction.

Understanding Gastritis

Gastritis is stomach lining inflammation, and it can bring discomfort and challenges to daily life. However, through mindful dietary choices and wholesome cooking, you can create meals that soothe and nourish, easing symptoms and promoting overall wellness.

Navigating Gastritis with Nutrition

Central to this cookbook is the belief that food is not only sustenance; it's medicine. By focusing on ingredients that are gentle on the stomach and crafting balanced, nutrient-rich dishes, we aim to empower individuals with gastritis to reclaim a good relationship with food in a healing and delicious way.

Creating Gastritis-Friendly Recipes

Each recipe has been meticulously crafted, drawing from a blend of culinary expertise and nutritional knowledge. Emphasizing whole, unprocessed foods, we've curated a collection that promotes digestive ease without compromising taste, so each dish brings joy to the table.

The Joy of Wholesome Eating

Our mission is to transform the perception of gastritis-friendly meals from a sacrifice of taste in the name of comfort to a celebration of nourishing, flavorful cooking. These recipes aren't simply about managing symptoms; they're about savoring every bite, knowing it contributes to both your enjoyment and your well-being.

Join us on this delicious journey toward gastritis management through mindful, wholesome eating. Let these recipes nurture your body and delight your senses, proving that healing and indulgence can coexist on your plate.

7 WAYS I DEAL WITH GASTRITIS

1. I don't drink coffee.

Coffee, naturally acidic, can irritate the stomach lining. By avoiding coffee, you are less likely to trigger the discomfort and inflammation associated with gastritis. Minimizing coffee intake helps maintain a more balanced pH environment in the stomach, contributing to digestive comfort.

2. I don't drink alcohol.

Alcohol can be harsh on the digestive system, leading to irritation and inflammation. Abstaining from alcohol keeps you from exacerbating gastritis symptoms and supports a healthier gut. Alcohol avoidance also allows the stomach to heal more effectively during gastritis recovery.

3. I stay away from spicy food.

Spicy foods can be a common trigger for gastritis symptoms. Avoiding spicy dishes helps prevent irritation and discomfort in the stomach lining. It also creates a soothing environment for your digestive system, minimizing the risk of inflammation.

4. I curb my sweet tooth.

Excessive sugar intake can contribute to inflammation and disrupt the balance of gut microbiota. Limiting sugary foods helps maintain a more stable environment in the digestive tract, so curb your sweet tooth to support overall gut health and reduce the likelihood of aggravating gastritis symptoms.

5. I don't eat fast food.

Fast food is often high in fat, salt, and additives, which can be challenging for the digestive system to process. Opting for whole, unprocessed foods over fast food prevents unnecessary stress on the stomach and intestines, supports better digestion and nutrient absorption, and reduces the risk of gastric irritation.

6. I don't overeat.

Overeating places additional strain on the digestive organs, potentially leading to discomfort and reflux. Practicing portion control helps the stomach process food more efficiently and provides your digestive system with a manageable workload, which promotes better digestion and minimizes the risk of gastritis flare-ups.

7. I'm mindful of my gut.

Being mindful of your gut involves paying attention to how your body responds to different foods and situations. Listening to signals of discomfort and adjusting your lifestyle accordingly supports ongoing gut health and allows you to make informed choices that align with your digestive well-being, fostering a proactive and holistic approach to managing gastritis.

Incorporating these practices into your daily life demonstrates a commitment to maintaining a healthy gut and managing gastritis effectively. Remember to always pay attention to your body's signals and make adjustments as needed.

Note on seasoning: Feel free to adjust the seasoning to your preferences. I've left out salt on a number of recipes and you can certainly curtail the amount to your personal taste.

Each recipe in this book is accompanied by fundamental notes, thoughtful suggestions, and valuable recommendations regarding nutritional benefits, enhanced nutrient content, and the chef's expert advice.

NB   **Nutritional Benefits**

EN   **Enhanced Nutrients/Improvements**

C   **Chefs Recommendation**

CHAPTER 1
Breakfast

Breakfast is essential to managing gastritis for several reasons.

Balances Blood Sugar

A healthy breakfast helps stabilize blood sugar levels, which is essential for individuals with gastritis. Stable blood sugar levels can prevent spikes that might aggravate symptoms like nausea or discomfort.

Prevents Excessive Stomach Acid

A nutritious breakfast, especially one that includes complex carbohydrates and proteins, can help buffer stomach acid, which reduces the chances of excess acid production that could irritate the stomach lining.

Provides Energy for the Day

A well-rounded breakfast provides essential nutrients and energy. For individuals managing gastritis, this energy can help sustain them throughout the day, minimizing the likelihood of feeling fatigued or overly hungry, which might aggravate symptoms.

Supports Medication Absorption

Eating breakfast can support the absorption of certain morning medications, as some drugs require food for optimal effectiveness. It also minimizes the risk of irritation to the stomach lining.

Choosing gastritis-friendly breakfast options like oatmeal, yogurt with non-citrus fruits, smoothies with mild ingredients, or eggs with whole-grain toast can be beneficial. Always tailor breakfast choices based on individual sensitivities and preferences to ensure they are gentle on the stomach and provide adequate nutrition to start the day on a positive note.

Quinoa Breakfast Bowl

1-2 servings

Ingredients:

- 1 cup cooked quinoa
- 1/2 cup almond milk
- 1 tablespoon maple syrup
- Toppings: sliced bananas, berries, chopped nuts

Instructions:

1) In a saucepan, warm cooked quinoa with almond milk and maple syrup until heated through.
2) Serve in a bowl, topped with sliced bananas, berries, and chopped nuts.

NB

- *Quinoa:* High in protein, fiber, and various nutrients like magnesium and iron.
- *Almond Milk:* Low in calories, high in vitamins and minerals like calcium and vitamin E.
- *Berries:* Rich in antioxidants, vitamins, and fiber.

EN

Consider adding a tablespoon of ground flaxseed or hemp hearts to boost omega-3 fatty acids and fiber and add nutrients without altering the taste.

C

Layer the quinoa, fruits, and nuts in a parfait glass or bowl for an aesthetically pleasing presentation. Garnish with mint leaves for a pop of color.

Chia Seed Pudding

1 serving

Ingredients:

- 1/4 cup chia seeds
- 1 cup coconut milk
  (or another plant based
  beverage)
- 1 tablespoon honey or agave syrup
- Toppings: Fresh fruits, shredded coconut

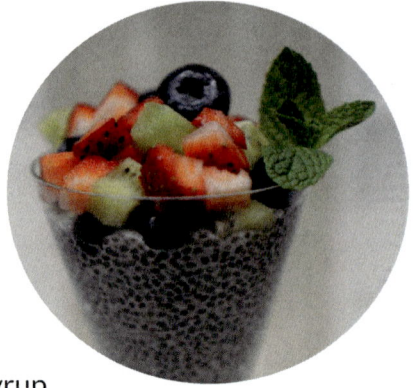

Instructions:

1) Mix chia seeds, coconut milk, and sweetener in a bowl.
2) Refrigerate for at least 2 hours or overnight until it thickens.
3) Serve with fresh fruits and shredded coconut on top.

NB

- *Chia seeds:* High in fiber, omega-3 fatty acids, protein, and various micronutrients.
- *Coconut milk:* Contains healthy fats and some vitamins and minerals.
- *Fresh fruits:* Provide vitamins, minerals, and antioxidants.

EN

Introduce a teaspoon of spirulina or matcha powder to the pudding mix for an added antioxidant boost and vibrant color.

C

Incorporate a crunchy element like toasted coconut flakes or chopped nuts as a topping for textural contrast and added flavor.

Buckwheat Pancakes

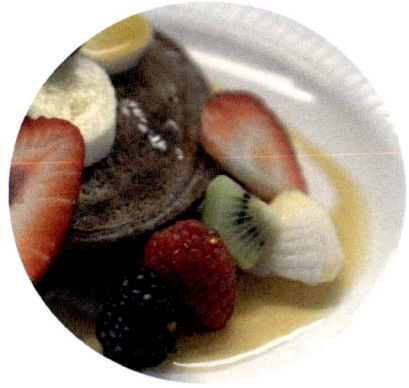

1 serving

Ingredients:

- 1 cup buckwheat flour
- 1 tablespoon coconut sugar
- 1 teaspoon baking powder
- 1 cup almond milk

Instructions:

1) In a bowl, mix buckwheat flour, coconut sugar, and baking powder.
2) Gradually add almond milk, whisk until smooth or until it resembles a batter consistency. If's it to thick add a teaspoon at a time of more almonds milk.
3) Cook pancakes on a non-stick pan until golden brown about 2 minutes for each side. Keep close eye on them that they don't get to brown

NB

- *Buckwheat flour:* Gluten-free, high in fiber, protein, and essential nutrients like manganese and magnesium.
- *Almond milk:* Low in calories, high in vitamins and minerals.

EN

Consider incorporating a plant-based protein powder or serving the pancakes with a side of almond butter for an additional protein kick.

C

Experiment with fresh fruit compotes or homemade fruit syrups to complement buckwheat's nutty flavor and elevate the overall taste profile.

Coconut Flour Banana Muffins

1-2 Servings

Ingredients:

- 1 cup coconut flour
- 1 teaspoon baking soda
- 3 ripe bananas, mashed (these need to be very ripe)
- 1/4 cup maple syrup
- 1/4 cup coconut oil, melted
- Coconut milk as needed.
- Pan spray

Instructions:

- Preheat the oven to 350°F (175°C) and line a muffin tin with liners. Use pan spray on the inside of the liners.
- In a bowl, mix coconut flour and baking soda. Add mashed bananas, maple syrup, and melted coconut oil. Stir until combined. If it's to dry try adding coconut milk a teaspoon at a time to reach the consistency of muffin batter.
- Pour batter into muffin cups and bake for 20-25 minutes or until a tooth pick inserted comes out clean.

NB

- *Coconut flour:* Gluten-free, high in fiber, and low in carbohydrates.
- *Ripe bananas:* Provide vitamins, potassium, and fiber.
- *Coconut oil:* Contains healthy fats with potential health benefits.

EN

Include a tablespoon of ground psyllium husk or whole oats to increase fiber content, aid digestion, and promote satiety.

C

Mix in a handful of dairy-free dark chocolate chips or chopped nuts to add texture and richness.

Sweet Potato Hash

2 Servings

Ingredients:

- 2 tablespoons olive oil
- 1 onion, diced
- 2 sweet potatoes, peeled and grated
- 1 teaspoon paprika
- Salt and pepper to taste if desired

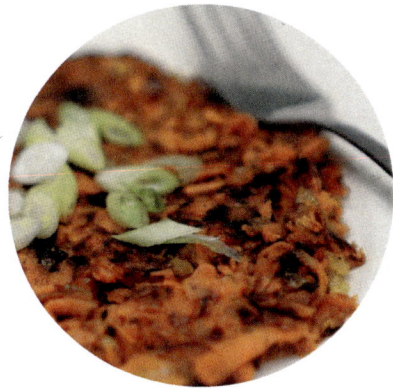

Instructions:

1) Heat olive oil to medium in a skillet. Add onions and cook until translucent.
2) Add grated sweet potatoes and paprika. Season with salt and pepper if desired.
3) Cook until potatoes are tender and slightly crispy about 5-8 minutes for each side. Keep an eye them they don't burn on the bottom and adjust the time for each side accordingly.

NB

- *Sweet potatoes:* High in vitamins A and C, potassium, fiber, and antioxidants.
- *Olive oil:* Contains healthy fats and antioxidants.

EN

Consider adding a sprinkle of ground ginger or turmeric for their anti-inflammatory properties, to support digestive health.

C

Incorporate fresh herbs like rosemary or thyme to enhance the flavor profile and add aromatic depth.

Avocado Toast with Poached Eggs

1 Serving

Ingredients:

- 2 slices gluten-free bread
- 1 ripe avocado
- 2 eggs
- Salt and pepper if desired

Instructions:

1) Toast the bread slices.
2) Mash avocado and spread it on the toast.
3) Poach eggs and place them on top of the avocado, making sure to dab the eggs with a paper towel or clean cloth. Sprinkle with salt and pepper if desired.

NB

- *Avocado:* Contains healthy fats, fiber, vitamins, and minerals.
- *Eggs:* High-quality protein, various vitamins, and minerals.

EN

Drizzle the avocado with a little apple cider vinegar. Its acidity has potential digestive benefits.

C

Experiment with different seasoning blends (e.g., za'atar, chili flakes, or smoked paprika) to add complexity.

Berry Smoothie Bowl

1 Serving

Ingredients:

- 1 cup mixed berries (frozen or fresh)
- 1/2 banana
- 1/2 cup almond milk
- Toppings: Granola, sliced fruits, shredded coconut

Instructions:

1) Blend mixed berries, banana, and almond milk until smooth.
2) Pour into a bowl and add toppings of choice.
3) Add more almond milk as needed to reach the desired consistency.

NB

- *Berries:* Rich in antioxidants, vitamins, and fiber.
- *Almond milk:* Low in calories, high in vitamins and minerals.
- *Granola:* Provides fiber, healthy fats, and some micronutrients.

EN

Incorporate a tablespoon of acai powder or a handful of spinach to enhance the smoothie's nutritional content.

C

Top the bowl with edible flower petals or a sprinkle of bee pollen for a visually appealing and sophisticated finish.

Tofu Scramble

2 Servings

Ingredients:

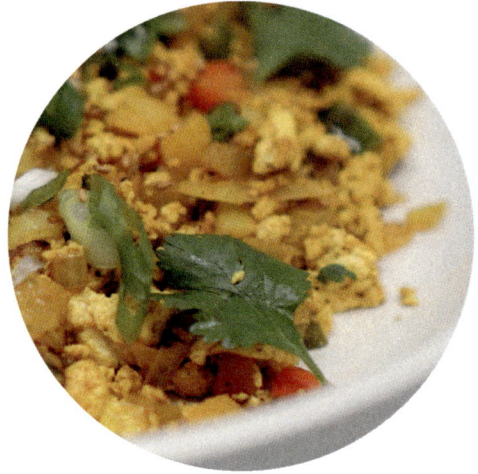

- 1 tablespoon oil
- 1/2 onion, diced
- 1 block firm tofu, crumbled
- 1 bell pepper, diced
- 1 teaspoon turmeric
- Salt and pepper to taste

Instructions:

1) In a skillet, over medium heat, add the oil.
2) When oil is hot, carefully add the onions and bell pepper, sauté until soft.
3) Add crumbled tofu and turmeric. Cook until tofu is heated through. Season with salt and pepper.

📋 NB

- *Tofu:* Good source of plant-based protein, iron, and calcium.
- *Vegetables:* Provide vitamins, minerals, and antioxidants.

🍏 EN Veggie Power

Increase the vegetable content by adding diced spinach, kale, or bell peppers for an extra nutrient boost.

🍽 C Flavor Infusion

Experiment with different spice blends or fresh herbs to add depth and complexity.

Cauliflower Breakfast Hash

2-4 Serving

Ingredients:

- 2 tablespoons olive oil
- 2 cups petite size ¼ to ½ inch cauliflower florets
- 1 red bell pepper, ¼ inch diced
- 1 small zucchini, ¼ inch diced
- 1 teaspoon smoked paprika
- Salt free seasoning or salt and pepper as desired

Instructions:

- In a skillet over medium heat olive oil until hot.
- Gently add cauliflower, bell pepper, and zucchini. Cook until vegetables are tender.
- Sprinkle with smoked paprika, add salt and pepper if desired.

NB

- *Cauliflower:* Low in calories, high in vitamins C and K, and a good source of fiber.
- *Bell pepper and zucchini:* Provide vitamins, minerals, and antioxidants.

EN

Sprinkle with a pinch of cinnamon or turmeric for their potential anti-inflammatory properties.

C

Introduce a handful of toasted seeds (such as pumpkin or sunflower seeds) for a delightful crunch to contrast the soft cauliflower.

Green Smoothie

1 serving

Ingredients:

- 1 cup spinach
- 1/2 cup pineapple chunks
- 1/2 cucumber, chopped
- 1 tablespoon chia seeds
- 1 cup coconut water- plus more as needed

Instructions:

1) Blend spinach, pineapple, cucumber, chia seeds, and coconut water until smooth. If it's too thick add a tablespoon at a time more coconut water until you reached the desired consistency

NB

- *Spinach:* Rich in vitamins A, C, K, and folate, and a good source of iron and antioxidants.
- *Pineapple and cucumber:* Provide vitamins, minerals, and hydration.
- *Chia seeds:* High in fiber, omega-3 fatty acids, and some minerals.

EN

Blend in a tablespoon of hemp seeds or ¼ - ½ cup silken tofu for added protein content to aid satiety and muscle repair.

C

Top the smoothie with a spiraled cucumber ribbon or a sprinkle of matcha powder for an elegant presentation.

CHAPTER 2
Lunch

Nutrient Intake and Healing

When dealing with or recovering from gastritis, a well-balanced, nutritious diet is imperative to support the healing process. A healthy lunch provides a variety of essential vitamins, minerals, and proteins that help repair and regenerate the stomach lining. Including lean proteins, whole grains, and a variety of fruits and vegetables in your lunch can contribute to a balanced diet and aid in the restoration of optimal digestive health.

Regular Meal Patterns and Stabilizing Blood Sugar Levels

Consistent meal patterns, including a nutritious lunch, play a key role in stabilizing blood sugar levels. Irregular eating habits (such as skipping meals) can lead to blood sugar fluctuations, which may exacerbate gastritis symptoms. Lunch is an important midday meal that helps maintain steady energy levels throughout the day, preventing prolonged periods of hunger that could contribute to stomach lining irritation. By stabilizing blood sugar, lunch supports overall wellness and promotes a more comfortable experience for individuals dealing with or recovering from gastritis.

Avoiding Aggravating Foods and Portions

When preparing your lunch, choose foods that are gentle on the stomach and avoid those that may exacerbate gastritis symptoms. Opting for smaller, more frequent meals during lunchtime can be beneficial, as large, heavy meals may put additional strain on the digestive system. Choosing easily-digestible options like soups, lean proteins, and cooked vegetables can minimize stomach lining irritation. By being purposeful about food choices and portion sizes, you can help manage and alleviate gastritis symptoms and promote a more comfortable recovery process.

Quinoa and Veggie Bowl

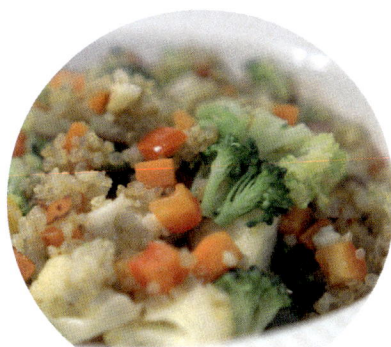

1-2 servings

Ingredients:

- 1 cup cooked quinoa
- 1 cup mixed veggies (broccoli, carrots, bell peppers, etc. cut up so they'll finish cooking about the same time)
- 1 tablespoon olive oil
- 1 clove garlic, minced
- Salt and pepper to taste

Instructions:

1) In a skillet over med-high heat, sauté veggies in olive oil until tender 5 minutes or until desired density is reached.
2) Add garlic and cook for another 20-30 seconds taking care not to burn the garlic.
3) Mix in cooked quinoa and remove from heat
4) Season to taste with salt and pepper.

NB

- *Quinoa:* Provides fiber for gut health.
- *Veggies:* Offer a variety of vitamins and minerals.

EN

Add a handful of chopped spinach for extra fiber.

C

Drizzle with lemon juice for added freshness.

Salmon and Avocado Wrap

1 serving

Ingredients:

- 4 oz. grilled salmon (flaked)
- 1 whole grain wrap
- 1/2 avocado, sliced
- 1 cup mixed greens
- 1 tablespoon Greek yogurt

Instructions:

1) Slightly warm the whole grain wrap in a pan over medium heat, remove the warp to a clean work surface.
2) Place the flaked salmon, avocado, and greens on the wrap.
3) Drizzle with Greek yogurt.
4) Wrap tightly like a burrito and enjoy.

NB

- *Salmon:* Provides omega-3 fatty acids.
- *Avocado:* Rich in healthy fats.

EN

Add a sprinkle of chia seeds for extra omega-3.

C

Add some crushed toasted cashews for extra crunch

Chickpea and Spinach Salad

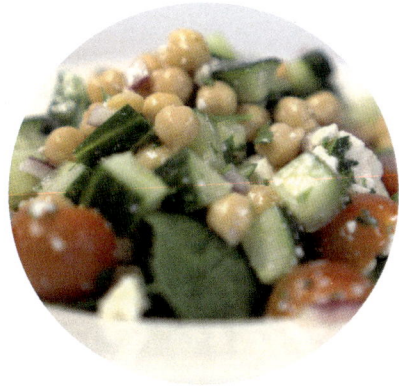

2 servings

Ingredients:

- 1 can chickpeas, drained and rinsed
- 2 cups fresh spinach
- 1/2 cup cherry tomatoes, washed and halved
- 1/4 cup feta cheese, crumbled
- 2 tablespoons balsamic vinaigrette

Instructions:

1) Combine chickpeas, spinach, tomatoes, and feta.
2) Drizzle with balsamic vinaigrette and toss to combine. Divide into two bowls and enjoy.

📋 NB

- *Chickpeas:* Provide plant-based protein.
- *Spinach:* High in iron and fiber.

🍎 EN

Toss in some sliced almonds for added vitamin e and manganese.

🍽 C

Add a pinch of dried oregano for flavor.

Yogurt-Tahini Dip with Vegetables

1 serving

Ingredients:

- 1 cup plain yogurt (low-fat or non-fat)
- 2 tablespoons tahini
- 1 clove garlic, minced
- 1 tablespoon lemon juice
- Salt and pepper to taste
- Assorted raw vegetables for dipping (carrots, cucumbers, bell peppers, etc.)

Instructions:

1) In a bowl, whisk together the plain yogurt, tahini, minced garlic, and lemon juice until smooth.
2) Season with salt and pepper to taste.
3) Serve the yogurt-tahini dip with assorted raw vegetables

NB

Low fat yogurt: Provides probiotics.

EN

Include a tablespoon of flaxseed for added fiber.

C

Cut the vegetable into fancy shape to create a visual enhancement.

Turkey and Quinoa Stuffed Peppers

4 servings

Ingredients:

- 2 bell peppers, halved
- 1/2 lb. ground turkey
- 1 cup cooked quinoa
- 1 cup tomato sauce
- 1 teaspoon Italian seasoning
- Salt and pepper as desired

Instructions:

1) Preheat the oven to 350 degrees.
2) Brown turkey until no longer pink about 8-10 minutes
3) Mixed the cooked turkey with cooked quinoa, the Italian seasoning and season with salt and pepper to desired preference.
4) Cool the mixture for 30 minutes.
5) Fill pepper halves; top with tomato sauce.
6) Bake for 30-40 minutes or until peppers are tender.

NB

- *Turkey:* Lean protein source.
- *Quinoa:* Provides fiber and essential amino acids.

EN

Add diced zucchini to the turkey mix for a good source of vitamins C and B6, as well as a variety of minerals, including potassium and manganese.

C

Garnish with fresh basil before serving.

Miso Soup with Tofu and Vegetables

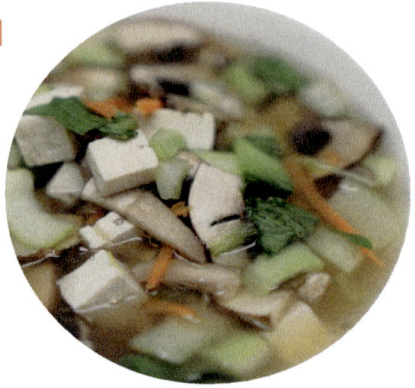

2-4 servings

Ingredients:

- 2 tablespoons miso paste
- 4 cups vegetable broth
- 1/2 cup tofu, cubed
- 1 cup mixed vegetables chopped small enough to fit onto a spoon. (bok choy, mushrooms, etc.)

Instructions:

1) In a large saucepan over medium heat, dissolve miso in vegetable broth.
2) Add tofu and veggies, simmer until cooked, do not boil soup.

NB

- *Miso:* Provides probiotics.
- *Tofu:* A good source of plant-based protein.

EN

Include seaweed for added minerals.

C

Sprinkle with green onions for freshness.

Sweet Potato and Lentil Soup

2 servings

Ingredients:

- 1 onion, chopped ¼ inch
- 2 cloves garlic, minced
- 1 large sweet potato, cubed ¼
- 1 tablespoon olive oil
- 1 cup dried lentils, rinsed
- 1 teaspoon cumin
- 4 cups vegetable broth
- Salt and pepper to taste

Instructions:

1) In a large pan over medium heat, add the olive oil.
2) When the oil is hot carefully add the onion and garlic and sauté until onions become translucent about 3-5 minutes, adjusting the heat being mindful not burn the garlic.
3) Add sweet potato, lentils, cumin, and broth.
4) Simmer until lentils are tender 12-15 minutes or until lentils are tender and not crunchy.
5) Season as desired with salt and pepper to taste.

NB

- *Sweet potatoes:* High in fiber and vitamins.
- *Lentils:* Provide plant-based protein.

EN

Stir in a handful of kale which is particularly notable for its exceptionally high levels of vitamin K, vitamin A, and vitamin C.

C

Finish with a squeeze of lemon for freshness.

Shrimp and Asparagus Stir-Fry

2 servings

Ingredients:

- 1/2 lb. shrimp, peeled and deveined
- 1 bunch asparagus, trimmed and cut into half inch pieces
- 1 bell pepper, sliced
- 1 tablespoon coconut oil
- 2 tablespoons soy sauce
- 1 tablespoon sesame oil
- 1 teaspoon fresh ginger, grated

Instructions:

1) Heat a large sauté pan over medium high heat.
2) Add 1 tablespoon coconut oil and stir-fry shrimp, asparagus, and bell pepper.
3) Mix in soy sauce, sesame oil, and ginger.

NB

- *Shrimp:* A low-calorie protein source.
- *Asparagus:* Provides fiber and antioxidants.

EN

Add a handful of snap peas for a good source of essential vitamins and rich in dietary fiber.

C

Garnish with sesame seeds for texture.

Cauliflower Rice Bowl with Black Beans

2-4 servings

Ingredients:

- 2 cups cauliflower rice
- 1 can black beans, drained and rinsed
- 1 cup corn kernels
- 1/2 cup salsa
- 1 avocado, sliced
- Salt and pepper as desired

Instructions:

1) Cook cauliflower rice according to package directions.
2) Mix with black beans, corn, and salsa.
3) Seasoning to taste with salt and pepper
4) Top with avocado slices.

NB

- *Cauliflower rice:* A low-carb rice alternative.
- *Black beans:* Provide fiber and protein.

EN

Add diced tomatoes for extra vitamins.

C

Squeeze lime juice over the bowl for an acidic tang.

Mediterranean Quinoa Salad

2 servings

Ingredients:

- 1 cup cooked quinoa
- 1/2 cucumber, ¼ diced
- 1 cup cherry tomatoes, halved
- 1/4 cup Kalamata olives, sliced in half
- 1/4 cup feta cheese, crumbled
- 2 tablespoons olive oil
- 1 tablespoon red wine vinegar
- Fresh basil, chopped

Instructions:

1) Combine quinoa, cucumber, tomatoes, olives, and feta.
2) Whisk together olive oil and red wine vinegar.
3) Toss salad with dressing.
4) Adjust seasoning to taste with salt and pepper if desired.
5) Garnish with basil.

NB

- *Quinoa:* Rich in fiber and essential amino acids.
- *Olive oil:* Provides healthy fats.

EN

Add chopped artichoke hearts as a good source of dietary fiber and antioxidants.

C

Serve chilled for a refreshing experience.

Chicken and Broccoli Casserole

2-4 servings

Ingredients:

- 2 cups cooked chicken, shredded
- 2 cups broccoli florets
- 1 cup quinoa, cooked
- 1 cup Greek yogurt
- 1/2 cup shredded cheddar cheese
- 1 teaspoon garlic powder
- Salt and pepper to taste
- Chicken stock as needed

Instructions:

1) Preheat the oven to 350 degrees
2) Mix chicken, broccoli, quinoa, Greek yogurt, and seasonings.
3) If the mixture is to thick, add a teaspoon at a time of chicken stock to loosen it up.
4) Transfer to a baking dish, top with cheddar cheese.
5) Bake for 30-40 minutes or until cheese is melted and bubbly.

NB

- *Chicken:* Good source of lean protein.
- *Greek yogurt:* Provides probiotics.

EN

Add diced red bell pepper for extra vitamins.

C

Sprinkle on chopped parsley for a burst of freshness.

Turmeric-Lemon Roasted Cauliflower

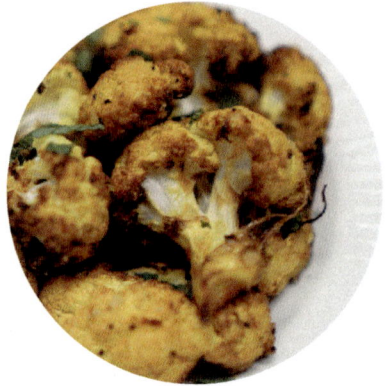

2-3 servings

Ingredients:

- 1 head cauliflower, cut into florets
- 3 tablespoons olive oil
- 1 teaspoon ground turmeric
- Zest of 1 lemon
- 2 cloves garlic, minced
- Salt and pepper to taste
- 1/4 cup chopped fresh parsley, for garnish

Instructions:

1) Preheat the oven to 400°F (200°C).
2) In a bowl, add the olive oil, ground turmeric, lemon zest and garlic- mix well.
3) Add the cauliflower florets and tossed until well combined.
4) Spread the cauliflower on a baking sheet in one layer and roast for 18-22 minutes until golden brown, check on them after 10 minutes and keep an eye on them so they do not burn.
5) Garnish with fresh parsley before serving.

NB

- *Cauliflower:* Rich in fiber and antioxidants.
- *Turmeric:* Anti-inflammatory properties.
- *Lemon:* Vitamin C and digestive aid.

EN

Sprinkle with flaxseed for added omega-3 fatty acids.

C

Serve as a flavorful side dish or over quinoa for a complete meal.

CHAPTER THREE
Dinner

Having a healthy dinner is beneficial for gut wellness, especially for individuals suffering from gastritis, for several reasons:

Reduced Irritation

Gastritis is inflammation of the stomach lining. Certain foods, such as those high in fat, spice, and acidity, can irritate the stomach lining and exacerbate symptoms. A healthy dinner typically includes foods that are gentle on the stomach, reducing irritation and discomfort.

Nutrient-Rich Foods

A well-balanced and healthy dinner includes a variety of nutrient-rich foods, such as fruits, vegetables, lean proteins, and whole grains. These foods provide essential vitamins, minerals, antioxidants, and fiber that support overall digestive health and can aid in the healing process.

Maintaining a healthy microbiome is crucial for digestive health, and this involves fostering a diverse and balanced gut microbiome. Consuming a variety of fiber-rich foods promotes the growth of beneficial bacteria in the gut, helping to maintain a healthy balance of microorganisms. This, in turn, supports the immune system and reduces inflammation associated with gastritis.

Balancing Acidity

Acidic foods and beverages can aggravate gastritis symptoms. A healthy dinner often includes alkaline-forming foods, such as leafy greens and certain fruits, which can help balance stomach acidity and reduce irritation.

Avoiding trigger foods is crucial for individuals with gastritis, as they frequently have specific foods that exacerbate their symptoms A healthy dinner plan involves avoiding these triggers, which can vary from person to person. Common triggers include spicy foods, caffeine, alcohol, and highly acidic foods.

Promoting Healing

Certain nutrients, such as zinc, vitamin A, vitamin C, and omega-3 fatty acids, play a role in the healing of the stomach lining. Including foods rich in these nutrients can support the healing process for individuals with gastritis.

Regulating portion sizes is essential, as overeating can impose additional stress on the stomach lining and exacerbate gastritis symptoms. A healthy dinner typically involves appropriate portion sizes to avoid overloading the digestive system.

It's important to note that individual responses to foods can vary, and what works well for one person may not be suitable for another. It's advisable for individuals with gastritis to work closely with a healthcare professional or a registered dietitian to create a personalized and effective dietary plan based on their specific needs and tolerances.

Salmon and Quinoa Bowl

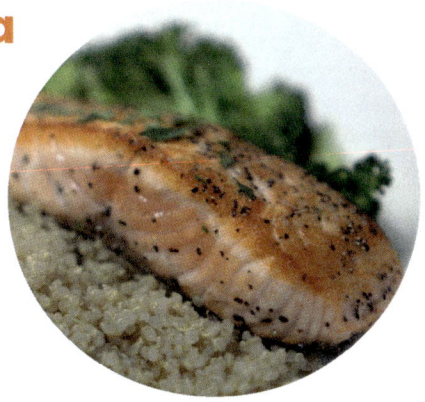

1 serving

Ingredients:

- 1 cup cooked quinoa
- 6 oz. grilled salmon
- 1 cup steamed broccoli florets
- 1 tablespoon olive oil
- Lemon wedges for garnish
- Seasoning to taste with favorite seasoning or salt and pepper to desired taste.

Instructions:

1) Arrange quinoa, salmon, and broccoli in a bowl.
2) Season as desired.
3) Drizzle with olive oil.
4) Garnish with lemon wedges.

NB

- *Salmon:* Provides omega-3 fatty acids.
- *Quinoa:* Offers fiber and essential amino acids.

EN

Add a side of sautéed kale for some key nutrients including vitamins A, K, C and B6.

C

Sprinkle with dill for a burst of flavor.

Vegetable Stir-Fry with Tofu

1-2 servings

Ingredients:

- 1/2 cup firm tofu, cubed
- 2 cups mixed vegetables (bell peppers, carrots, snap peas, etc. cut to size so they finish cooking at the same time.)
- 1 tablespoon sesame oil
- 1 tablespoon soy sauce
- 1 teaspoon fresh ginger, minced
- Brown rice

Instructions:

1) Sauté tofu and vegetables in sesame oil.
2) Add soy sauce and ginger.
3) Serve over brown rice.

NB

- *Tofu:* Provides plant-based protein.
- *Mixed vegetables:* Offer vitamins and fiber.

EN

Include broccoli which is rich content of vitamins, minerals, fiber, and various bioactive compounds.

C

Drizzle with a touch of chili oil for heat.

Lentil and Vegetable Soup

1-2 servings

Ingredients:

- 1 cup dried green lentils, rinsed
- 2 carrots, ¼ inch diced
- 2 celery stalks, ¼ inch diced
- 1 small onion, ¼ inch chopped
- 4 cups vegetable broth
- 1 teaspoon cumin
- Salt and pepper to taste

Instructions:

1) In a saucepan, combine lentils, carrots, celery, onion, and broth.
2) Add cumin, salt, and pepper.
3) Simmer for about 20 minutes or until lentils are tender.

NB

- *Lentils:* Provide protein and fiber.
- *Vegetables:* Offer a variety of vitamins.

EN

Stir in a handful of spinach which is high in vitamins, an excellent source of minerals and high in antioxidant.

C

Finish with a squeeze of lemon for a brighter flavor.

Mushroom and Spinach Quiche

4 servings

Ingredients:

- 1 pre-made whole wheat pie crust
- 1 tablespoon olive oil
- 1 cup mushrooms, sliced
- 2 cups fresh spinach
- 4 eggs
- 1 cup milk (or non-dairy alternative)
- 1/2 cup feta cheese, crumbled

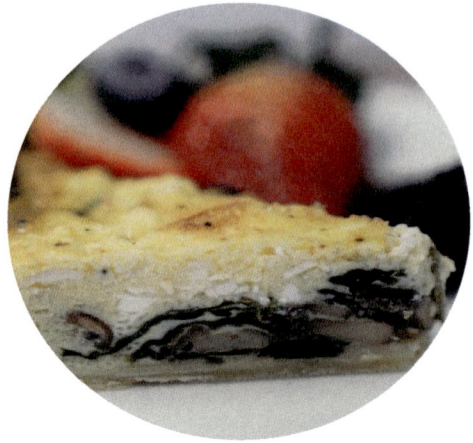

Instructions:

1) Preheat the oven to 350 degrees.
2) In a skillet, over medium heat add the olive oil and sauté mushrooms until soft then add the spinach until wilted and remove from heat and let cool for about 5-10 minutes.
3) Whisk together eggs and milk.
4) Mix sautéed mushroom and spinach into the pie crust. Then add the milk and egg mixture then pour over the veggies and into the quiche base.
5) Season lightly, if desired with salt and pepper
6) Top with feta.
7) Bake for 40-50 minutes or until set.

🗒️ NB

- *Spinach:* Provides iron and fiber.
- *Eggs:* Offer protein and essential nutrients.

🥗 EN

Add diced tomatoes which are relatively low in calories, making them a healthy and nutrient-dense addition to various meals.

🍽️ C

Garnish with fresh herbs like parsley or chives.

Chickpea and Sweet Potato Curry

2-4 servings

Ingredients:

- 1 can chickpeas, drained and rinsed
- 2 sweet potatoes, peeled and diced ¼ inch size
- 1 tablespoon olive oil
- 1 onion, chopped ¼ inch size
- 2 cloves garlic, minced
- 1 can coconut milk
- 2 tablespoons curry powder
- Basmati rice

Instructions:

1) In a skillet, over medium high heat add the olive oil.
2) Sauté onion and garlic until onions are soft.
3) Add sweet potatoes and chickpeas.
4) Stir in curry powder and coconut milk.
5) Simmer for 10 minutes or until sweet potatoes are tender, add more liquid if necessary.
6) Taste and adjust the seasoning with salt and pepper if desired.

NB

- *Chickpeas:* Provide protein and fiber.
- *Sweet potatoes:* Offer vitamins and antioxidants.

EN

Include a handful of kale which contains vitamins like A, K and C.

C

Serve over basmati rice with a squeeze of lime.

Turkey and Vegetable Skewers

2-4 servings

Ingredients:

- 1 lb. turkey breast, cut into cubes 1 inch cubes
- 1 Bell peppers, 1 inch cubes
- 1 pint cherry tomatoes,
- 1 large zucchini, cut into chunks 1 inch size
- 2 tablespoons olive oil
- 1 teaspoon dried oregano
- Salt and pepper to taste

Instructions:

1) Thread turkey and veggies onto skewers.
2) Mix olive oil, oregano, salt, and pepper.
3) Brush skewers with the mixture.
4) Grill and medium high heat for about 3-5 minutes per side. Depending on how thick the cubes are and how hot the grill is. Turkey is cooked when it reaches an internal temperature of 165 degrees.
5) Make sure to let the turkey and vegetable skewers rest for 3-5 minutes before eating.

NB

- *Turkey:* Lean protein source.
- *Vegetables:* Provide vitamins and fiber.

EN

Add a handful of spinach to serve kabobs on which is rich in vitamins, minerals, fiber, and antioxidants.

C

Serve with a side of tzatziki for a Mediterranean twist.

Quinoa and Black Bean Stuffed Peppers

4 servings

Ingredients:

- 4 bell peppers, halved
- 1 cup cooked quinoa
- 1 can black beans, drained and rinsed
- 1 cup corn kernels
- 1 cup salsa
- 1 teaspoon cumin

Instructions:

1) Preheat the oven to 350 degrees.
2) In a mixing bowl, combine quinoa, black beans, corn, salsa, and cumin.
3) Add your favorite seasoning to taste or salt and pepper to taste.
4) Fill pepper halves with the mixture. Place in an oven proof casserole style dish.
5) Bake for 34-40 minutes or until peppers are tender.

NB

- *Quinoa:* Provides fiber and essential amino acids.
- *Black beans:* Offer protein and fiber.

EN

Top with diced avocado are an excellent source of dietary fiber. Fiber promotes digestive health, helps maintain a feeling of fullness, and supports stable blood sugar levels.

C

Sprinkle with cilantro before serving.

Grilled Lemon Herb Chicken

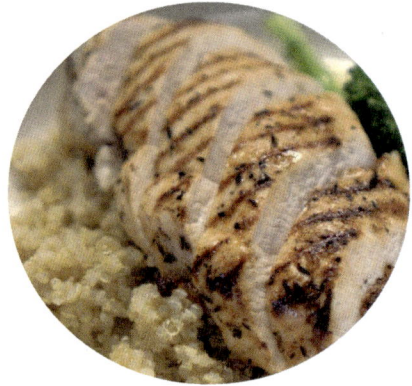

4 servings

Ingredients:

- 4 boneless, skinless chicken breasts
- 2 lemons, juiced
- 2 tablespoons olive oil
- 1 teaspoon dried thyme
- Salt and pepper to taste

Instructions:

1) Mix lemon juice, olive oil, thyme, salt, and pepper.
2) Marinate chicken in the mixture for 30 minutes.
3) Grill Chicken for about 5 minutes per side or until fully cooked. The internal temperature reached 165 degrees.

NB

- *Chicken:* Source of lean protein.
- *Lemon:* Provides vitamin C.

EN

Create a sauce using Greek yogurt, lemon juice, garlic and herbs, a creamy, tangy topping that adds protein and probiotics.

C

Serve with a side of roasted Brussels sprouts.

Baked Cod with Tomato and Olive Salsa

4 servings

Ingredients:

- 4 cod fillets
- 1 cup cherry tomatoes, halved
- 1/4 cup Kalamata olives, sliced in half
- 2 tablespoons olive oil
- 1 tablespoon balsamic vinegar
- Salt and pepper to desired taste

Instructions:

1) Preheat the oven to 350 degrees.
2) Place cod fillets on an oil casserole style oven proof container.
3) Mix tomatoes, olives, olive oil, and balsamic vinegar.
4) Season to taste for personal perferences
5) Spoon the salsa over the cod and bake for about 8 minutes or until fish flakes.

NB

- *Cod:* Low-fat protein source.
- *Tomatoes and olives:* Offer antioxidants.

EN

Add a handful of arugula to the salsa which is a good source of dietary fiber,

C

Garnish with a sprinkle of feta cheese.

Pesto Zucchini Noodles with Grilled Shrimp

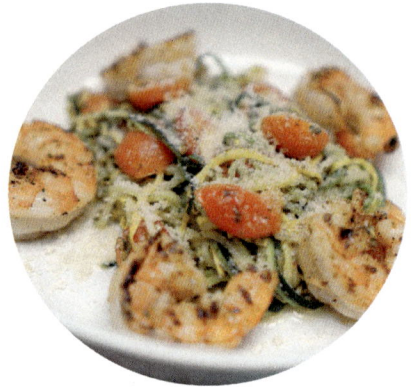

4 servings

Ingredients:

- 1 lb. shrimp, peeled and deveined
- 4 medium zucchinis, spiraled
- 1/2 cup cherry tomatoes, halved
- 1 tablespoon olive oil
- 1/4 cup pesto sauce
- 2 tablespoons grated Parmesan cheese

Instructions:

1) Grill shrimp for two minutes or until cooked. Internal temperature should reach 145 degrees according to the USDA
2) In a skillet, over medium high heat add the olive oil.
3) Sauté zucchini noodles until tender.
4) Drain off any excess water from the zucchini.
5) Toss noodles with cherry tomatoes, pesto, and shrimp.
6) Season accordingly and to personal preference.
7) Top with Parmesan cheese.

📋 NB

- *Shrimp:* Provides lean protein.
- *Zucchini:* Low-calorie, hydrating vegetable.

🍎 EN

Mix in cooked chickpeas or white beans for extra fiber and proteins.

🍽 C

Squeeze fresh lemon juice over the dish before serving.

Eggplant and Chickpea Curry

2-4 servings

Ingredients:

- 1 onion, ¼ inch chopped
- 2 cloves garlic, minced
- 1 large eggplant, ¼ cubed
- 1 can chickpeas, drained and rinsed
- 1 can diced tomatoes
- 1 tablespoon olive oil
- 2 tablespoons curry powder
- 1/2 cup coconut milk
- Basmati rice

Instructions:

1) In a skillet, over medium high heat add the olive oil.
2) Sauté onion and garlic until softened.
3) Add eggplant, chickpeas, tomatoes, and curry powder.
4) Pour in coconut milk. Simmer for about 15 minutes or until eggplant is tender.
5) Season to taste with salt and pepper if desired

NB

- *Eggplant:* Provides fiber and antioxidants.
- *Chickpeas:* Offer protein and fiber.

EN

Elevate the nutritional content by gently folding in a generous handful of finely chopped cilantro just before serving, infusing the dish with additional vitamins, including A, K, and C

C

Serve over basmati rice with a side of naan.

Turkey and Vegetable Stir-Fry

2-4 servings

Ingredients:

- 1/2 lb. ground turkey
- 1 teaspoon sesame oil
- 2 cups broccoli florets
- 1 bell pepper, sliced
- 1 cup snap peas
- 2 tablespoons soy sauce
- 1 tablespoon hoisin sauce
- Chicken stock as needed

Instructions:

1) In a skillet, brown turkey in sesame oil for about 10 minute or until all the ground turkey is cooked and there is no pink.
2) Add veggies, soy sauce, and hoisin sauce.
3) Add a tablespoon at a time of chicken stock to help keep the stir-fry from burning on the bottom.
4) Stir-fry until veggies are tender.

NB

- *Turkey:* Lean protein source.
- *Vegetables:* Provide vitamins and fiber.

EN

Add sliced water chestnuts which are low in calories, a good source of carbohydrates and dietary fiber.

C

Garnish with toasted sesame seeds.

Spinach and Feta Stuffed Chicken Breast

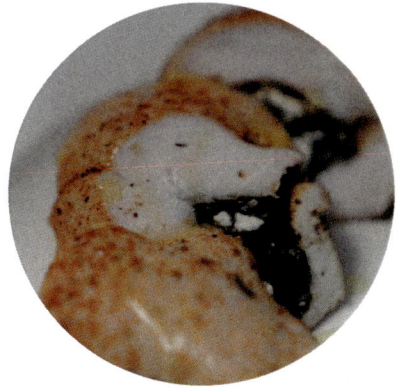

4 servings

Ingredients:

- 2 cups fresh spinach
- 1 clove garlic, minced
- 1 tablespoon chicken stock
- 1/2 cup feta cheese, crumbled
- 4 boneless, skinless chicken breasts
- Salt and pepper to taste if desired

Instructions:

1) Preheat the oven to 350 degrees.
2) In a skillet, over medium heat add the chicken stock.
3) Sauté spinach until wilted and water evaporated.
4) Remove from heat and mix in feta cheese, let the mixture cool for about 10 minutes.
5) Cut a pocket into the side of each chicken breast using a sharp thin knife, stuff with spinach mixture.
6) Bake for about 20-25 minutes or until chicken is cooked through and reaches a temperature of 165 degrees.

NB

- *Spinach:* Provides iron and fiber.
- *Chicken:* Lean source of protein.

EN

Sprinkle chopped nuts (such as almonds or walnuts) or seeds (like pumpkin or sunflower seeds) for added texture, healthy fats, and nutrients.

C

Sprinkle with fresh basil before serving.

Cauliflower and Chickpea Curry Bowl

2-3 servings

Ingredients:

- 1 onion, chopped ¼ inch size
- 2 cloves garlic, minced
- 1-2 tablespoon olive oil
- 1 head cauliflower, cut into florets
- 1 can chickpeas, drained and rinsed
- 2 tablespoons curry powder
- 1 can coconut milk
- Salt and pepper to taste
- Brown rice

Instructions:

1) In a skillet, over med-heat add the olive oil and sauté onion and garlic for about 3-5 or until softened.
2) Add cauliflower, chickpeas, curry powder, and coconut milk.
3) Simmer until cauliflower is tender.
4) Taste and adjust the seasoning as desired

NB

- *Cauliflower:* Provides fiber and antioxidants.
- *Chickpeas:* Offer protein and fiber.

EN

Mix in diced bell peppers for added vitamin C. Bell peppers are rich in vitamin C, which is a powerful antioxidant that supports the immune system, helps the body absorb iron, and promotes healthy skin.

C

Serve over brown rice with a squeeze of lime.

Sesame Ginger Tofu Stir-Fry

1-2 servings

Ingredients

- 1 tablespoon sesame oil
- 1/2 lb. firm tofu, cubed ½ inch size
- 2 cups mixed vegetables (broccoli, carrots, bell peppers, etc. ½ inch in size)
- 2 tablespoons soy sauce
- 1 tablespoon rice vinegar
- 1 teaspoon fresh ginger, grated
- Vegetable stock as needed
- Brown rice

Instructions:

1) In a skillet, over medium heat sauté tofu and vegetables in sesame oil.
2) Mix together soy sauce, rice vinegar, and grated ginger.
3) Pour soy sauce mixture over tofu and veggies. Stir-fry until heated through.
4) Add a tablespoon at a time of vegetable stock as needed to keep it saucy

NB

- *Tofu:* Provides plant-based protein.
- *Mixed vegetables:* Offer vitamins and fiber.

EN

Add bok choy, which is a cruciferous vegetable, belonging to the same family as broccoli and cabbage. These vegetables are known for their potential health benefits, including anti-inflammatory and anti-cancer properties.

C

Garnish with crushed toasted cashews for extra crunch and a sprinkle of thinly sliced green onions for color.

Thai In-spired Bean Salad

3-4 servings

Ingredients:

- 1 can chickpeas, drained and rinsed
- 1 can black beans, drained and rinsed
- 1 cucumber, diced ¼ inch
- 1 cup cherry tomatoes, halved
- 1 carrot, grated
- ½ cup chopped cilantro
- ¼ cup sliced green onions
- ¼ cup chopped peanuts or cashews
- ¼ cup chopped Thai basil for garnish

For the dressing

- ½ cup fresh lime juice or mild vinegar such as rice, add smaller amounts when converting until desired flavor is reached.
- 2 tablespoon tamari or soy sauce
- 2 tablespoon sesame oil
- 1 tablespoon honey or maple syrup
- 1 tablespoon grated ginger
- 2 clove garlic minced
- Salt and pepper to taste

Instructions:

1) In a large bowl combine the first seven ingredients.
2) Whisk together the dressing ingredients.
3) Toss salad with half the dressing and then increase until you've reached the desired texture, garnish with chopped nuts and basil.

NB

- *Chickpeas:* Provide protein and fiber.
- *Vegetables:* Offer a variety of vitamins.

EN

Add chopped sweet peppers for a high source of antioxidants

C

Serve as a side or with grilled chicken for a complete meal.

Mango and Black Bean Quinoa Salad

2 servings

Ingredients:

- 1 cup cooked quinoa
- 1 can black beans, drained and rinsed
- 1 ripe mango, ¼ diced
- 1/2 red onion, chopped 1/8 inch
- 1/4 cup cilantro, chopped
- 2 tablespoons lime juice
- 2 tablespoons olive oil
- Salt and pepper to taste

Instructions:

1) Combine quinoa, black beans, mango, red onion, and cilantro.
2) Whisk together lime juice, olive oil, salt, and pepper.
3) Toss salad with dressing.
4) Taste and adjust for seasoning accordingly

NB

- *Quinoa:* Provides fiber and essential amino acids.
- *Black beans:* Offer protein and fiber.
- *Mango:* Provides vitamins and antioxidants.

EN

Add a handful of arugula for extra leafy greens which boost minerals like iron, calcium, magnesium and potassium.

C

Toasted pumpkin seeds make a great crunchy topping.

Teriyaki Chicken and Broccoli Stir-Fry

2-4 servings

Ingredients:

- 1 lb. chicken breasts, sliced thin
- 2 cups broccoli florets
- 1 carrot, julienned
- 1 tablespoon sesame oil
- 1/4 cup teriyaki sauce
- 2 tablespoons soy sauce
- 1 tablespoon honey
- Vegetable stock as needed
- Brown rice

Instructions:

1) In a skillet, on medium high heat stir-fry chicken, broccoli, and carrot in sesame oil for 6-8 minutes or until chicken is fully cooked. Chicken is done at 165 degrees.
2) Mix together teriyaki sauce, soy sauce, and honey.
3) Pour sauce over stir-fry. Cook until heated through.
4) Add a teaspoon at a time of vegetable stock if sauce it too thick.
5) Taste and adjust seasoning as desired

NB

- *Chicken:* Lean source of protein.
- *Broccoli:* Provides vitamins and fiber.
- *Teriyaki sauce:* Adds flavor without excessive calories.

EN

Include shiitake mushrooms are a good source of B-vitamins, including B2 (riboflavin), B5 (pantothenic acid), and B6 (pyridoxine). They also contain minerals such as copper, selenium, and zinc. Additionally, shiitake mushrooms are known for their potential immune-boosting and anti-inflammatory properties.

C

Garnish with sesame seeds for texture.

Lemon Herb Grilled Tofu Skewers

2 servings

Ingredients:

- 1/2 lb. firm tofu, 1 inch cubed
- 1 zucchini, sliced 1 inch thick
- 1 yellow bell pepper, 1 inch square
- 2 tablespoons olive oil
- 1 lemon, juiced and zested
- 1 teaspoon dried thyme
- Salt and pepper to taste

Instructions:

1) Thread tofu, zucchini, and bell pepper onto skewers.
2) Mix together olive oil, lemon juice, lemon zest, thyme, salt, and pepper.
3) Brush skewers with the seasoning mixture.
4) Grill over med-high heat on each side for 2-3 minutes or until tofu is golden. Keep a close eye on them to prevent them from burning

NB

- *Tofu:* Provides plant-based protein.
- *Zucchini:* Offers vitamins and antioxidants.
- *Lemon:* Adds vitamin C.

EN

Marinate tofu in a balsamic-herb mixture which would help to keep low calories and providing a flavorful addition.

C

Serve over a bed of quinoa for a complete meal.

Caprese Stuffed Portobello Mushrooms

4 servings

Ingredients:

- 4 large Portobello mushrooms
- 1 cup cherry tomatoes, halved
- 1/2 cup fresh mozzarella, diced
- 1/4 cup fresh basil, chopped
- 2 tablespoons balsamic glaze
- 2 tablespoons olive oil
- Salt and pepper to taste

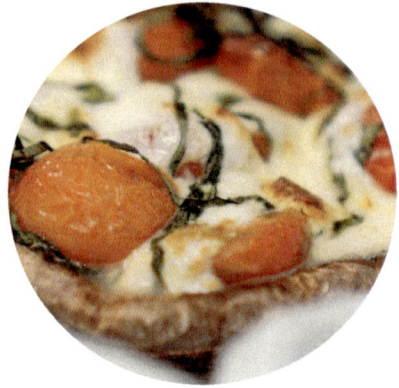

Instructions:

1) Preheat oven to 400.
2) Remove stems from mushrooms. Brush with olive oil.
3) Combine tomatoes, mozzarella, and basil.
4) Stuff mushroom caps.
5) Bake for 6-12 minutes or until mushrooms are tender.
6) Drain excess moisture from tomatoes if necessary,
7) Drizzle with balsamic glaze before serving.
8) Season to taste as desired

NB

- *Portobello mushrooms:* Low in calories and rich in antioxidants.
- *Tomatoes:* Provide vitamins and lycopene.
- *Fresh mozzarella:* Adds protein and calcium.

EN

Mix in diced artichoke hearts for Prebiotics. Artichokes contain inulin, a type of prebiotic fiber that can promote the growth of beneficial gut bacteria. This can contribute to a healthy gut microbiome.

C

Drizzle with a basil-infused olive oil for extra aroma.

Coconut-Curry Chickpea Bowl

2 servings

Ingredients:

- 2 cans chickpeas, drained and rinsed
- 1 cup cauliflower florets
- 1 cup snow peas
- 1 tablespoon olive oil
- 1 can coconut milk
- 1-2 teaspoon red curry paste (be mindful of spice level)
- 1 tablespoon soy sauce or tamari
- Vegetable stock as needed
- Cooked jasmine rice

Instructions:

1) In a skillet, over medium heat add the olive oil.
2) Sauté chickpeas, cauliflower, and snow peas in red curry paste.
3) If need be you can add a tablespoon of vegetable stock to prevent any stickiness to the pan
4) Add coconut milk and soy sauce. Simmer until veggies are tender.
5) Serve over jasmine rice.

NB

- *Chickpeas:* Provide protein and fiber.
- *Cauliflower:* Offers vitamins and antioxidants.
- *Coconut milk:* Adds healthy fats.

EN

Include spinach for added iron and folate.

C

Top with chopped cilantro for freshness.

CHAPTER 4
Dessert

For people going through and recovering from gastritis, dessert recipes can actually play a significant role in supporting the healing process, for three practical reasons.

Comfort and Satisfaction

Recovering from gastritis sometimes involves dietary restrictions and a bland meal plan. Desserts provide a source of comfort and satisfaction, making the overall eating experience more enjoyable. Feeling satisfied and enjoying meals can help alleviate stress and promote a positive mindset, which contributes to overall well-being during recovery.

Nutrient-Dense Ingredients

Well-designed dessert recipes—like the ones in this book—incorporate nutrient-dense ingredients that offer essential vitamins and minerals. For example, fruits, nuts, and certain sweeteners can provide nutritional benefits.

Including nutrient-dense desserts in your diet ensures that the body receives necessary nutrients for healing without compromising on taste. This approach is particularly important, as the gastritis diet may limit certain food choices.

Maintaining Social Connections

Desserts are often associated with social gatherings and celebrations, so indulging in dessert allows individuals with gastritis to participate in social events without feeling left out.

Maintaining social connections is important for emotional wellness. Desserts provide an opportunity for individuals to share a meal with others from start to finish, which contributes to a sense of normalcy and support during the recovery process.

Note

It's essential to tailor dessert recipes to individual dietary needs and preferences, avoiding ingredients that may trigger or exacerbate gastritis symptoms. Opting for low-acid fruits and non-acidic sweeteners and avoiding spicy or overly-rich ingredients can help create desserts that are gentle on the stomach.

Always consult with a healthcare professional or a registered dietitian to ensure that dessert choices align with specific dietary recommendations during gastritis recovery.

Probiotic Berry Parfait

2 servings

Ingredients:

- 1 cup Greek yogurt
- 1/2 cup mixed berries (blueberries, strawberries, etc.)
- 1/4 cup granola
- 1 tablespoon honey

Instructions:

1) In a glass, layer Greek yogurt, berries, and granola.
2) Drizzle with honey.

NB

- *Greek yogurt:* Provides probiotics for gut health.
- *Berries:* Rich in antioxidants.

EN

Add a tablespoon of chia seeds for extra fiber.

C

Garnish with mint leaves for freshness.

Banana "Nice Cream"

4 servings

Ingredients:

- 4 ripe bananas, peeled, sliced, and frozen
- 1/4 cup dairy-free milk (such as almond milk, coconut milk, or oat milk)
- Optional toppings: crushed nuts, cinnamon, honey (if tolerated)

Instructions:

1) Place the frozen banana slices in a blender or food processor.
2) Add the dairy-free milk to the blender.
3) Blend the mixture on high until smooth and creamy, stopping occasionally to scrape down the sides of the blender if needed. If the mixture is too thick, you can add a little more dairy-free milk, but be careful not to add too much, as you want the nice cream to be thick and creamy.
4) Once the nice cream reaches a smooth consistency, it is ready to serve. If you prefer a softer texture, you can enjoy it immediately as soft-serve nice cream.
5) If you prefer a firmer texture, transfer the nice cream to a container and freeze it for about 30 minutes to 1 hour.
6) When ready to serve, scoop the nice cream into bowls and top with your favorite toppings, such as crushed nuts, a sprinkle of cinnamon, or a drizzle of honey if tolerated.
7) Serve immediately and enjoy!

NB

- *Bananas:* Offer potassium and prebiotics.

EN

Include a tablespoon of ground flaxseed for omega-3.

C

Add shredded coconut for added texture

Mango-Coconut Tapioca Pudding

2 servings

Ingredients:

- 1/4 cup small tapioca pearls
- 1 cup coconut milk (use light coconut milk if preferred or other plant-based beverage)
- 1 ripe mango peeled and diced.
- 1-2 tablespoons honey or maple syrup (adjust to taste)
- A pinch of salt

Instructions:

1. Prepare Tapioca Pearls:

Rinse the tapioca pearls under cold water in a fine-mesh strainer. Drain well.

2. Soak Tapioca Pearls:

In a small bowl, cover the tapioca pearls with water and let them soak for about 15-20 minutes. This helps soften them before cooking.

3. Cook Tapioca Pearls:

In a small saucepan, combine the soaked tapioca pearls, coconut milk, and a pinch of salt over medium heat. Stir occasionally to prevent sticking.

Bring the mixture to a gentle simmer, then reduce the heat to low. Let it simmer for about 10-15 minutes or until the tapioca pearls turn translucent and become soft, stirring occasionally.

4. Sweeten:

Once the tapioca pearls are cooked, add honey or maple syrup to sweeten the pudding, adjusting to your taste preference. Stir well to incorporate.

5. Blend Mango:

In a blender or food processor, puree the diced mango until smooth. You can add a splash of water if needed to help blend.

6. Combine Mango Puree:

Pour the mango puree into the cooked tapioca pudding mixture. Stir well until thoroughly combined.

7. Chill:

Remove the saucepan from heat and let the pudding cool slightly. Then transfer it to the refrigerator to chill for at least 1-2 hours, or until cold.

8. Serve:

Once chilled, divide the mango-coconut tapioca pudding into serving bowls. You can garnish with sliced almonds, shredded coconut, or fresh mint leaves if desired.

NB

Mango: Provides vitamins and digestive enzymes.

EN

Stir in a tablespoon of hemp seeds for extra protein.

C

Optional toppings: sliced almonds, shredded coconut, or fresh mint leaves for garnish.

Papaya Lime Sorbet

4 servings

Ingredients:

- 2 cups ripe papaya, cubed
- Juice of 2 limes
- 2 tablespoons honey
- Mint leaves for garnish

Instructions:

1) Blend papaya, lime juice, and honey until smooth.
2) Freeze for 4 hours, stirring every hour.
3) Scoop into bowls, garnish with mint.

NB

- *Papaya*: Contains digestive enzymes.
- *Lime:* Provides vitamin C.

EN

Add a tablespoon of grated ginger for anti-inflammatory benefits.

C

Serve with a wedge of lime for an extra burst of flavor.

Yogurt-Dipped Frozen Grapes

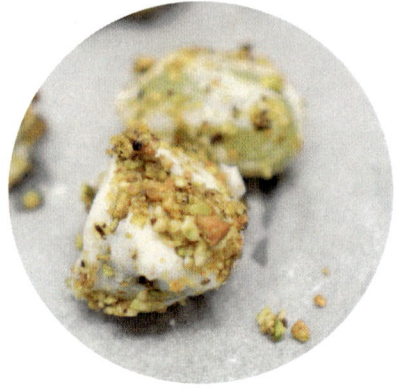

2 servings

Ingredients:

- 1 cup grapes (red or green)
- 1/2 cup plain Greek yogurt
- 1 tablespoon honey
- Chopped pistachios for coating

Instructions:

1) Dip grapes in Greek yogurt to coat them.
2) Place on a tray and freeze for 2 hours.
3) Drizzle with honey and roll in chopped pistachios.

📋 NB

1) *Greek yogurt:* Provides probiotics.
2) *Grapes:* Offer resveratrol and natural sweetness.

🍎 EN

Use a mix of colored grapes for a variety of antioxidants.

🛎 C

Sprinkle with a pinch of sea salt for a sweet-savory contrast.

These dessert recipes aim to be both delicious and supportive of gut health, but you should always adjust ingredients based on personal preferences and dietary restrictions. Enjoy the educational, entertaining, and fun experience of creating and indulging in these treats!

CONCLUSION

As we conclude this journey toward better gut health, I encourage you to make a personal commitment to prioritize your wellness. Remember, small changes lead to big results. Embrace the power of nourishing your gut, and may your path forward be a healthier, happier you be filled with vitality and joy.

Optimal gut wellness is a lifelong endeavor. As you close this book, remember that every dietary choice you make impacts your gut. Look ahead with optimism, knowing that each mindful decision contributes to a healthier you.

I want to express my deepest gratitude to you for joining me on this exploration of gut wellness. The digestive tract is a remarkable ecosystem, and your commitment to understanding and caring for it is commendable. As you continue your journey, remember that you're part of a community dedicated to health. Stay connected, share your successes, and inspire others to embark on their own gut health adventure.

In the words of Jim Rohn, "Your life does not get better by chance; it gets better by change." Your journey toward digestive wellness is no different. Take that step today, and let it be the start of a transformative and fulfilling path. Your entire being will thank you.

Made in the USA
Monee, IL
10 September 2025